Super Ramen Recipe Book for Beginners

Super Tasty, Quick and Easy Ramen Collection

Jonathan Rees

© **Copyright 2020 - All rights reserved.**

The content contained within this book may not be reproduced, duplicated or transmitted without direct written permission from the author or the publisher.

Under no circumstances will any blame or legal responsibility be held against the publisher, or author, for any damages, reparation, or monetary loss due to the information contained within this book. Either directly or indirectly.

Legal Notice:

This book is copyright protected. This book is only for personal use. You cannot amend, distribute, sell, use, quote or paraphrase any part, or the content within this book, without the consent of the author or publisher.

Disclaimer Notice:

Please note the information contained within this document is for educational and entertainment purposes only. All effort has been executed to present accurate, up to date, and reliable, complete information. No warranties of any kind are declared or implied. Readers acknowledge that the author is not engaging in the rendering of legal, financial, medical or professional advice. The content within this book has been derived from various sources. Please consult a licensed professional before attempting any techniques outlined in this book.

By reading this document, the reader agrees that under no circumstances is the author responsible for any losses, direct or indirect, which are incurred as a result of the use of information contained within this document, including, but not limited to, — errors, omissions, or inaccuracies.

Table of Contents

Peanut ramen 7

Fire ramen 10

Fish bowl 13

Shrimp Sriracha Ramen 15

Vegetable soup with tofu 18

Green peanut ramen 20

Meatball Ramen 23

Chicken fillet soup 25

Coconut curry (vegan) 27

Pumpkin and tomato soup 30

Swiss chard ramen 32

Mexican Chicken Ramen 34

Miso ramen (vegan) 37

Pak Choi ramen to go 39

Pak Choi Tofu Ramen (vegan) 41

Chicken ramen 43

Pulled beef stew 46

All sorts of ramen 49

Ramen Pho 51

Ramen to go 54

King prawn pot 56

Beef ramen 59

Pork tenderloin and spinach ramen 61

Pork ramen 64

Pork ramen soup 66

Summer soup 67

Bacon ramen 70

Tomato Ramen Soup 72

lemon grass soup 74

Banana split 76

Butterscotch shards 79

Ice cream ramen 81

Peanut Butter Bread 83

Peanut Butter Chocolate Ramen 85

Honey and cinnamon ramen 87

Crispy cherry ramen 89

Cereal bites 91

Peach ramen 93

Ramen cookies 95

Chocolate ramen 97

Chocolate bar 99

Chocolate vanilla ramen 101

Trail mix with honey 103

Walnut pile 105

Peanut ramen

for 4 servings

for 40 minutes

easily

ingredients

200 grams of snow peas

250 grams of mushrooms, brown

300 grams of ramen

2 liters of vegetable stock

1 teaspoon curry paste

2 tablespoons of coconut oil

2 tablespoons of miso paste

2 tablespoons of raw cane sugar

2 tablespoons of soy sauce

4 tablespoons of peanut butter

½ pointed cabbage

1 chili pepper, red

1 walnut-sized piece of ginger

1 lime

2 carrots

2 cloves of garlic

4 eggs

preparation

1 Wash the chili pepper thoroughly, halve and core it, and finely chop half of the chili. Peel the ginger and garlic and finely chop both. Heat the coconut oil in a large saucepan, add the chili, ginger and garlic and roast everything. Deglaze the contents of the pot with the soy sauce and stir in the curry paste, peanut butter, miso paste and sugar. Pour the vegetable stock over the pot and then let the soup simmer for about 17 minutes.

2 Meanwhile, cook the ramen al dente, pour them off and let them drain well. Cook the eggs in a small saucepan for about 6 minutes until they are waxy. Wash and clean the snow peas and cut them into strips. Peel the carrot and use a peeler to cut it into fine, long strips. Clean the pointed cabbage, cut it into strips and wash it off thoroughly. Clean the mushrooms, cut them in half if necessary, and then cut them into fine slices.

3 After 17 minutes, add the vegetables to the pot from step 1 and let the soup cook for another 3 minutes. Season the soup with the lime juice.

4 Divide the soup into 4 bowls and pour the broth over them. Peel the eggs, then cut them in half and serve them on the

soup. Cut the leftover chili into thin rings and garnish the soup with them.

Fire ramen

for 2 servings

less than 30 minutes

easily

ingredients

200 grams of ramen

1 liter of water

1 teaspoon vegetable stock

2 teaspoons of Sambal Oelek

2 teaspoons of sesame oil

2 teaspoons of tahini

1 tablespoon miso paste

1 tablespoon of olive oil

2 tablespoons of soy sauce

1 packet of dashi powder

1 dash of almond milk (almond drink)

1 carrot

1 onion

2 cloves of garlic

4 shiitake mushrooms, dried

some sesame

preparation

1 Soak the shiitake mushrooms in hot water for 5 minutes. Meanwhile, peel the onion and cut it into eighths. Peel the carrots and cut them diagonally into slices about 2 millimeters thick. Peel the garlic and press it down with the side of the knife.

2 Put some oil in a saucepan and heat it over medium heat. Then add the carrots, garlic, shiitake mushrooms and onions and fry them brown. This should create a s brownish layer on the bottom of the pot.

3 Smear the contents of the pan with the water and vegetable stock. Then stir in the dashi powder and miso paste, season and season to taste. Then let the soup simmer until the carrots are cooked through.

4 Meanwhile, cook the ramen al dente, pour them off and let them drain well.

5 Put 1 teaspoon each of the sambal oelek, 1 teaspoon of the sesame oil, 1 teaspoon of the sesame paste and 1 tablespoon of the soy sauce in small bowls and stir everything together thoroughly.

6 Remove the carrots and shiitake mushrooms from the soup and cut the mushrooms into strips for the garnish.

7 Stir a dash of milk into the soup. Then distribute this on the bowls and stir it with the liquid that is already there.

8 Put the ramen in the bowls and use a fork to twist them up in a spiral. Garnish with the carrot slices, the shiitake mushrooms and sprinkled with the sesame seeds before serving.

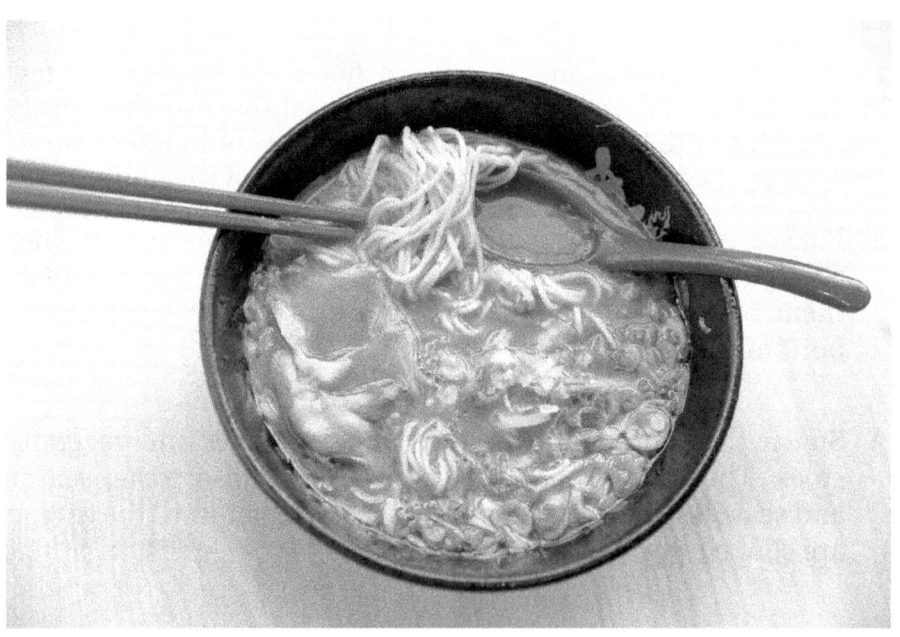

Fish bowl

for 10 servings

for 40 minutes

easily

ingredients

10 grams of chili, chopped

50 grams of spring onions, cut into rings

75 grams of sugar

200 grams of mung bean sprouts

200 grams of shiitake mushrooms, cut into strips

380 grams of ramen

40 milliliters of lime juice

50 milliliters of vegetable oil

120 milliliters of white wine

360 milliliters of soy sauce

10 redfish fillets

preparation

1 Mix the soy sauce, the white wine and the sugar with 2 liters of water until the sugar has completely dissolved, warming it up a little if necessary.

2 Boil the bouillon from step 1 with the chili, lime juice and mushrooms. Add the mung bean sprouts and ramen and let them steep for 5 minutes.

3 Brush the fish fillets with the vegetable oil and grill them all over. Then keep it warm.

4 Fill the soups into bowls and garnish each with 1 fish fillet. Spread the spring onions over the dish to serve.

Shrimp Sriracha Ramen

for 6 servings

less than30 minutes

easily

ingredients

20 grams of baby spinach leaves

250 grams of large shrimp, peeled, deveined

300 grams of ramen

300 milliliters of water

600 milliliters of chicken broth

½ teaspoon of garlic powder

½ teaspoon pepper

½ teaspoon of salt

½ teaspoon of celery salt

½ teaspoon onion powder

1 teaspoon basil, dried

1 teaspoon rice vinegar

1 tablespoon of ginger

1 ½ tablespoons of soy sauce

2 tablespoons of sriracha

2 tablespoons of tomato paste

2 tablespoons lemon juice, fresh

3 tablespoons of sesame oil

1 small bell pepper, red

1 small onion, yellow

6 cloves of garlic

preparation

1. Wash the baby spinach leaves and chop them roughly. Peel the ginger, garlic, and onion, finely grate the ginger, chop the garlic, and dice the onion. Wash the peppers thoroughly and cut them into cubes.

2. Put 1 tablespoon of the sesame oil in a large saucepan and heat over medium-high heat. Add the shrimp in a single layer, then sprinkle with the dried basil, pepper, and salt. Fry the prawns on each side for about 1 minute until they turn opaque. Take the prawns out of the pot and place them on a cutting board.

3. Put the remaining sesame oil in the same saucepan and heat it over medium heat. Then add the bell pepper, sriracha sauce and onion and cook for about 4 minutes, stirring occasionally. Then add the ginger and garlic and cook for 1 more minute.

4 Pour the contents of the pot on with the chicken stock and water and stir everything well. Turn up the heat and bring the soup to a boil. Then stir in the garlic powder, rice vinegar, celery salt, soy sauce, tomato paste and onion powder. Reduce the heat again and let the soup simmer for about 8 minutes.

5 In the meantime, cut the prawns into bite-sized pieces.

6 Add the ramen to the soup and cook them for 2 minutes while stirring. Then add the prawns, spinach and lemon juice and stir everything together again. Taste the soup and season it if necessary.

7 Divide the soup into bowls and serve immediately.

Vegetable soup with tofu

for 4 servings

for 60 minutes

easily

ingredients

10 grams of ginger

100 grams of spinach leaves

100 grams of mushrooms

100 grams of ramen noodles

100 grams of tofu

750 milliliters of vegetable broth

4 teaspoons of sesame oil, toasted

6 tablespoons soy sauce, light

1 clove of garlic

4 spring onions

pepper

salt

preparation

1 Peel the ginger and garlic, chop finely and mix both with the soy sauce. Cut the tofu into fine strips and turn it in the marinade.

2 Clean the spring onions, wash them thoroughly and cut them diagonally

into thin rings. Rub the mushrooms clean and cut them into slices. Pick the spinach leaves, wash them thoroughly and let them drain well.

3 Boil the broth in a wok, add the mushrooms and spring onions and let everything simmer for about 1 minute. Then add the ramen noodles and cook them for about 4 minutes.

4 Add the marinade, spinach and tofu to the wok and heat everything for another minute.

5 Season the soup with salt and pepper, divide it into bowls and drizzle with the sesame oil to serve.

Green peanut ramen

for 4 servings

for 40 minutes

easily

ingredients

80 grams of peanut butter

100 grams of green beans

130 grams of broccoli

200 grams of mushrooms, brown

250 grams of ramen

800 milliliters of vegetable broth

1 teaspoon chili flakes

2 teaspoons of curry powder

3 teaspoons of ginger, fresh

3 tablespoons of soy sauce

6 tablespoons of lime juice

1 can of coconut milk (400 milliliters)

1 handful of peanuts

2 spring onions

5 cloves of garlic

pepper

salt

preparation

1. Peel the ginger and garlic, then chop both finely. Put some oil in a saucepan, heat it and fry the ginger and garlic in it until they give off an intense scent.

2. Pour the contents of the pot on with the vegetable stock and coconut milk. Then add the chili flakes, the curry powder, the peanut butter, the lime juice and the soy sauce as a soup base, stir the whole thing well and let it boil. Then season the contents of the pot with salt and pepper.

3. Meanwhile, clean the mushrooms and cut them into slices. Wash the beans, broccoli, and green onions thoroughly. Cut the beans into bite-sized pieces, the broccoli into florets, and the spring onions into thin rings.

4. As soon as the soup base starts to boil in the pot, add the vegetables from step 3. Let this cook for another 5 minutes.

5 Then add the ramen and cook them al dente. Season the dish with lots of salt and pepper, divide it into bowls and garnish with peanuts for serving.

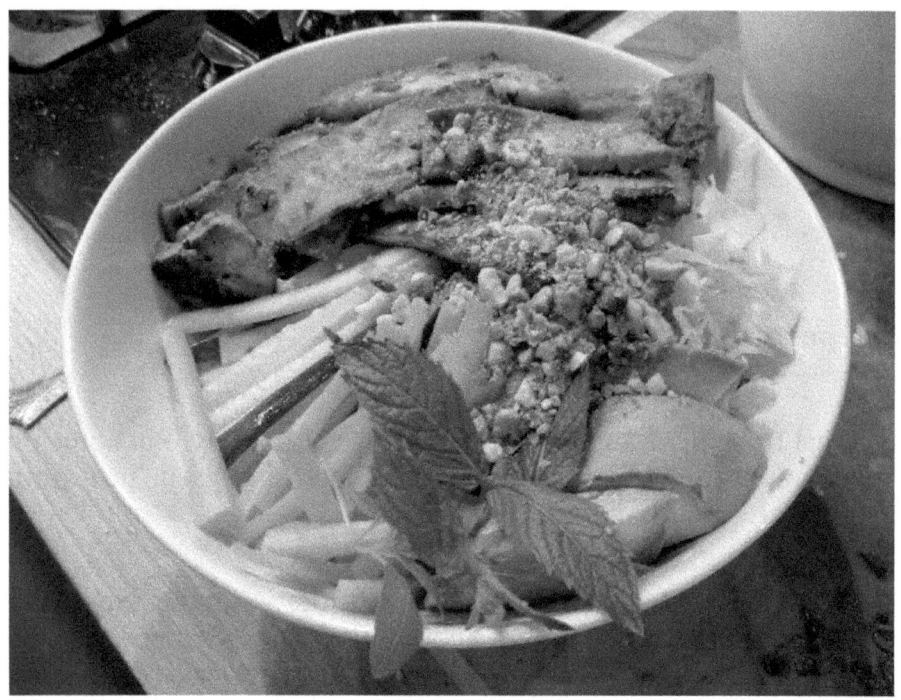

Meatball Ramen

for 4 servings

less than 30 minutes

easily

ingredients

270 grams of ramen

400 grams of ground beef

1 liter of dashi broth

2 tablespoons of miso paste

2 tablespoons of breadcrumbs

2 tablespoons of soy sauce

6 stalks of chives, cut into fine rolls

½ celery stalk, sliced

1 egg, size M

1 zucchini, donated

1 onion, diced pepper

salt

preparation

1. Mix the egg with the minced meat, breadcrumbs, soy sauce and onions. Season the mixture with pepper and salt and form about 20 small meatballs from it.

2. Cook the ramen for 4 minutes, then drain and drain well. Boil the broth, add the meatballs, celery and zucchini and cook for 10 minutes. Then mix the miso paste with some of the hot broth and stir it into the saucepan with the broth.

3. Add the ramen to the broth and divide the dish into bowls. Then serve it garnished with the chives.

Chicken fillet soup

for 2 servings

less than 30 minutes

easily

ingredients

80 grams of mung bean sprouts

80 grams of ramen

120 grams of chicken breast fillet

350 grams of chicken broth

1 teaspoon instant wakame

1 tablespoon of soy sauce

1 tablespoon of sunflower oil

2 tablespoons of miso, red

2-3 tablespoons of sweet chili sauce

5 centimeters of leek

1 carrot

1 clove of garlic

preparation

1. Cut the chicken breast fillet into narrow strips. Peel the garlic and chop it finely. Clean, peel and cut the carrot into sticks about two inches long. Halve the leek, wash it thoroughly and cut it lengthways into strips. Place the mung bean sprouts in a colander and rinse them thoroughly with cold water.

2. Boil the broth and add the carrots, leek, ramen and instant wakame. Let everything cook on medium heat for about 2 to 4 minutes and then add the mung bean sprouts - let everything steep.

3. Meanwhile, put the oil in the pan or in a wok and heat it up. Fry the chicken breast fillet strips and the garlic in them on high heat for about 1 minute. Then pour in the soy and sweet chili sauce and let the pan fry for another 2 minutes on medium heat.

4. Remove the pan from the stove and stir the miso paste into the soup. Divide these into bowls, fold in the meat and serve the soup.

Coconut curry (vegan)

for 6 servings

less than30 minutes

easily

ingredients

150 grams of sugar snap peas

200 grams of ramen

200 grams of shiitake mushrooms

1 liter of vegetable stock

2 teaspoons of curry powder

1 tablespoon of sesame oil

1-3 tablespoons of curry paste, red

1 small bunch of coriander

1 can of coconut milk (400 milliliters)

1 walnut-sized piece of ginger

1 lime

2 carrots

2 cloves of garlic Chili;

Limes

Hot peppers

pepper

salt

preparation

1 Peel the ginger, carrots and garlic, chop the ginger and garlic and cut the carrots into pens. Clean the shiitake mushrooms and cut them into slices. Wash the sugar snap peas and cut them diagonally into pieces. Squeeze out the lime.

2 Put the sesame oil in a large saucepan and heat it over medium heat. Then add the peas, carrots and shiitake mushrooms to the saucepan and steam everything, stirring occasionally, for about 3 to 4 minutes.

3 Add the curry paste, curry powder, chopped ginger and chopped garlic to the pot and stir-fry for about 1 minute.

4 Deglaze the contents of the pot with the vegetable stock and coconut milk and season to taste with salt and pepper. Then bring the contents of the pot to the boil and add the ramen. Cook the latter until they are firm to the bite.

5 Stir in the lime juice and divide the soup into bowls. Garnish the dish with chilies and fresh coriander and serve with split limes.

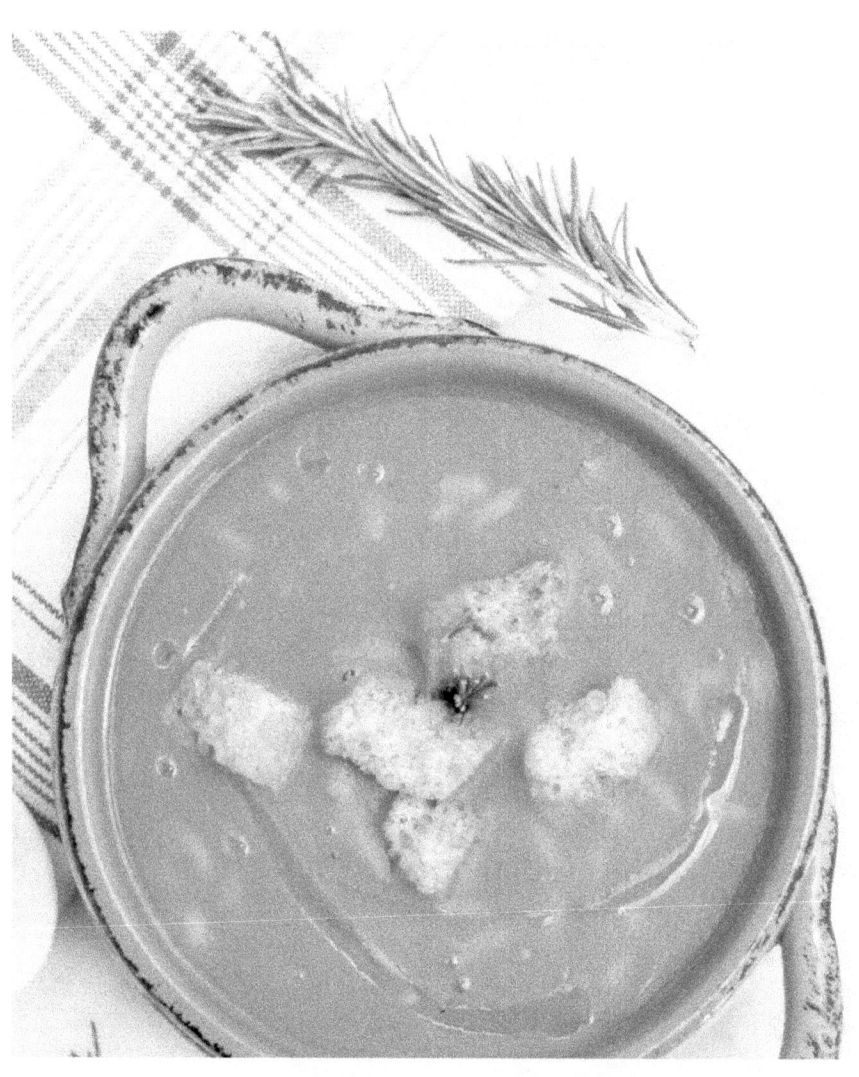

Pumpkin and tomato soup

for 8 servings

for 40 minutes

easily

ingredients

260 grams of ramen

400 grams of canned tomatoes, diced

480 grams of butternut squash, diced

150 milliliters of cream

900 milliliters of vegetable broth

½ teaspoon pepper, red, crushed

1 tablespoon of sage, chopped

1 tablespoon of thyme, chopped

2 tablespoons of olive oil

1 onion, diced

2 celery stalks, diced

3 cloves of garlic, chopped

For the garnish:

Pumpkin seeds, roasted

Cream Splatter

preparation

1   In a large saucepan, heat some oil over medium heat. Add the butternut squash, celery, and onions and cook for about 8 minutes.

2   Meanwhile, cook the ramen al dente, pour them off and let them drain well.

3   Add the garlic, pepper, sage and thyme to the saucepan with the pumpkin and cook the whole thing while stirring for 2 minutes.

4   Deglaze the contents of the pot with the vegetable stock and add the diced tomatoes. Boil the whole thing, reduce the heat and let the soup simmer for about 10 to 15 minutes until the butternut squash is soft.

5   Use a hand blender to puree the soup. Then stir in the cream, heat the soup again for 5 minutes, then season it to taste.

6   Divide the soup into bowls and add the ramen. Garnish the soup with the pumpkin seeds and the cream.

Swiss chard ramen

for 4 servings

for 30 minutes

easily

ingredients

20 grams of ginger, chopped

200 grams of Swiss chard, cut into thin strips

200 grams of shiitake mushrooms, sliced

250 grams of ramen

1 ½ liter of vegetable stock

4 tablespoons of soy sauce

1 can of corn

1 pinch of chili

2 carrots, cut into sticks

oil

preparation

1   Heat some oil in a wok. Fry the ginger, carrots, Swiss chard and shiitake mushrooms (without their stems) for about 5 minutes.

2   Meanwhile, cook the ramen in the vegetable stock with a pinch of chili for about 6 minutes. Add the vegetables from the wok and the corn and season the soup with the soy sauce.

3   Divide them into bowls and serve immediately.

Mexican Chicken Ramen

for 4 servings

for 40 minutes

easily

ingredients

120 grams of ramen

500 grams of chicken breast

600 milliliters of chicken broth

600 milliliters of water

¼ teaspoon of cayenne pepper

1 teaspoon of salt

2 teaspoons of chili powder

2 teaspoons of coriander

2 teaspoons of cumin

2 teaspoons of Mexican oregano, dried

1-2 tablespoons of oil

1 small can of chilies, green

1 lime, the juice of it

1 tomato

1 onion

4 cloves of garlic

optional ingredients

Avocado slices

spring onions

coriander

lime

sour cream

preparation

1   Cut the chicken breast into cubes. Peel the garlic and onion, coarsely chop the garlic, and dice the onion.

2   Heat 1-2 teaspoons of oil in a large pan and fry the onions until translucent. Add the meat and garlic and cook for 5 to 6 minutes, stirring, until the meat starts to brown.

3   Add the spices and oregano to the pan and cook for 1 minute. Then add the broth, the chili, the tomatoes and the water and cook everything over high heat.

4 Cook the ramen in it, reduce the heat and let the pan simmer for about 10 minutes until the ramen is cooked through.

5 Squeeze out the lime and season the contents of the pan with the lime juice and salt.

6 Divide the dish on bowls and garnish with avocado, spring onions, coriander and lime wedges.

Miso ramen (vegan)

for 2 servings

less than 30 minutes

easily

ingredients

50 grams of bean sprouts

100 grams of tofu for soups

100 grams of ramen

600 milliliters of vegetable broth

¼ teaspoon chili flakes

2 teaspoons of miso

1 tablespoon of oil, neutral

¼ nori sheet

2 spring onions

2 cloves of garlic

4 shiitake mushrooms, fresh or dried

preparation

1. Soak the dried shiitake mushrooms in a small amount of water for about ½ hour. Let the mushrooms boil briefly, then let them cool down and then cut them into strips. With fresh shiitake mushrooms, you can cut them directly into strips. Wash and clean the spring onions thoroughly, then cut them into fine rings. Cut the nori sheet into strips and dice the tofu.

2. Chop the garlic and put it in a pan with the vegetable oil. Fry the garlic in it and add the chili flakes and miso paste. Then remove the contents of the pan with the vegetable stock.

3. Cook the ramen al dente, then drain and drain well. Then divide them into bowls, fill the whole thing up with the miso broth and serve the dish with the spring onions, nori strips, shiitake mushrooms, bean sprouts and the tofu.

Pak Choi ramen to go

for 2 servings

less than 30 minutes

easily

ingredients

20 grams of ginger, chopped

50 grams of beef, cut into small pieces

90 grams of ramen

2 teaspoons of miso paste, dark

2-4 tablespoons of kimchi

6 stalks of coriander, roughly chopped

2 baby pak choi, cut into small pieces

2 cloves of garlic, chopped

4 spring onions, cut into rings

6 shiitake mushrooms, thinly sliced

salt

preparation

1 Cook the ramen al dente, then drain and drain well.

2 Place the ginger, kimchi, garlic, and miso paste in two mason jars and stir thoroughly.

3 Layer the ramen, pak choi, shiitake mushrooms, spring onions, meat and coriander on top.

4 To serve, pour boiling water over the whole thing, close the lid and let it steep for 5 minutes.

Pak Choi Tofu Ramen (vegan)

for 10 servings

ingredients

300 grams of ramen

400 grams of tofu

200 milliliters of soy milk

70 minutes easily2 liters of vegetable stock

2 tablespoons of coconut oil

3 tablespoons of soy sauce

4 tablespoons of miso paste

1 walnut-sized piece of ginger

1 chili pepper, red

2 onions, red

3 mini pak choi

4 spring onions

5 cloves of garlic

15 shiitake mushrooms

preparation

1 Wash the chili, core them and cut them into fine rings. Peel the ginger, garlic, and onion and chop roughly everything. Clean the mushrooms.

2 Heat 1 tablespoon of oil in a large saucepan and fry the chili, ginger, garlic and onion in it. Add the stock and 5 mushrooms and let everything simmer on low for about 1 hour.

3 Meanwhile, wash and clean the spring onions and the pak choi and cut the spring onions into thin rings and the pak choi into strips. Cut the remaining mushrooms into strips and the tofu into small cubes.

4 Cook the ramen al dente, then drain and drain well. Heat some oil in a pan and fry the tofu on all sides until crispy. Then deglaze it with the soy sauce.

5 Stir the miso paste and soy milk into the broth and simmer for another 5 minutes.

6 Arrange the vegetables and ramen in bowls, pour the stock over them and spread the tofu on top. Serve immediately.

Chicken ramen
for 4 servings

for 60 minutes

easily

ingredients

200 grams of chicken breast

250 grams of ramen

250 milliliters of water

300 milliliters of clear soup

2 tablespoons of miso paste

1 sheet of seaweed

1 handful of spinach leaves

2 handfuls of broccoli

1 chili pepper

1 large carrot

2 Eggs
2spring onions

Bamboo shoots

Coriander, fresh pepper

salt

soy sauce

preparation

1 Put the vegetable bouillon together with the miso paste, the seaweed leaf and the water in a large saucepan and cook everything for about 5 minutes.

2 Cut the chicken into slices about 1 centimeter thick and add them to the stock until it is cooked.

3 Wash the chili pepper thoroughly, cut it in half and remove the stone. Then add the chili to the pot and cook them too.

4 Cook the ramen al dente, then drain and drain well. Be careful not to let them get too soft, as they'll stick in the bouillon later.

5 Put the eggs in a small saucepan and cook them until they are waxy for about 6 minutes. Then frighten it off, peel it, and then cut it in half.

6 Wash the spinach and broccoli then cut the latter into bite-sized pieces. Wash the spring onions and cut them into thin strips. Wash the carrot, peel it, and cut it into fine slices.

7 Put the vegetables in the pot and let them cook until they are firm to the bite. Just before the end of the cooking time, add the spinach and season the dish with the pepper, salt and soy sauce.

8 Divide the ramen in bowls, pour the soup over them and garnish with the bamboo shoots, eggs and coriander.

Pulled beef stew

for 4 servings

for 60 minutes

easily

ingredients

100 grams of shiitake mushrooms

125 grams of mung bean sprouts

250 grams of ramen

2 liters of chicken stock

2 tablespoons of sesame oil

4 tablespoons of peanuts, salted

4 tablespoons of soy sauce

½ bunch of coriander

½ bunch of radishes

1 stick of lemongrass

1 spring onion

1 carrot

1 clove of garlic

1 red pepperoncini

1 pulled beef

2 shallots

4 eggs size M

preparation

1   Peel the clove of garlic and shallots. Finely chop the clove of garlic and cut the shallots into thin rings. Clean the shiitake mushrooms and cut them into strips. Wash the spring onions and lemongrass, cut the spring onions into thin rings, and finely chop the inside of the lemongrass. Peel the carrot and cut it into fine pencils.

2   Put the eggs in a small saucepan and cook them until they are waxy for about 6 minutes. Scare them off afterwards and let them cool down well.

3   Prepare the pulled beef according to the packaging instructions, pluck it apart and mix it with 3 tablespoons of the liquid from the bowl. Then warm up the pulled beef. Boil the bouillon.

4   Heat some oil in a pan and sauté all ingredients - with the exception of the lemongrass - for about 4 minutes. Pour in the bouillon and soy sauce and bring the pan to a boil. Then add the ramen and cook them al dente.

5   Spread the ramen including the soup in bowls and spread the vegetables on top. Scatter the peanuts on top and garnish the dish with sprigs of coriander.

All sorts of ramen

for 2 servings

for 30 minutes

ingredients

200 grams of ramen

1 liter of water, hot

4 level teaspoons of chicken broth

3 tablespoons of soy sauce

4 tablespoons of mirin

2 eggs

2 chicken breast fillets

2 cloves of garlic

2 pak choi

10 mushrooms or other mushrooms

some ginger

preparation

1 Mix the chicken broth with the hot water. Peel the ginger and the clove of garlic and cut both into small pieces. Heat the

mirin and soy sauce in a saucepan and add the ginger and clove of garlic.

2. Boil the egg in a small saucepan until it is waxy for about 6 minutes. Then chill the egg and let it cool completely in ice water. Then cut the egg in half lengthways. Cook the ramen in the chicken broth until al dente.

3. Pour the chicken broth with the ramen through a sieve into the saucepan with the ginger, garlic, mirin and soy sauce and mix well.

4. Cut the chicken breast fillet into slices about 1 centimeter thick and fry them in a little fat, mirin and soy sauce. Cut the pak choi and mushrooms into small pieces and sweat them too.

5. Put the ramen in small bowls and serve them together with the halved egg, the chicken breast fillet, the pak choi and the mushrooms and pour the broth over them.

Ramen Pho

for 2 servings for 60 minutes

ingredients

100 grams of ramen

600 milliliters of vegetable broth

¼ teaspoon pepper, red

½ teaspoon of Chinese five-spice powder

½ teaspoon fish sauce, optional

½ teaspoon sesame oil, toasted

1 teaspoon rapeseed oil

1 teaspoon sugar, light brown

2 teaspoons of soy sauce

1 tablespoon lime juice, fresh

1 piece of ginger

1 small onion

chicken

For the garnish (optional)

basil

halved waxy eggs

spring onions

Jalapeño

Coriander leaves

Lime wedges

mint

Onions

preparation

1   Peel the ginger and cut it in half lengthways. Peel the onion and cut it in half. Cut the meat into slices.

2   In a large saucepan, heat the oil over medium heat. Add the halved ginger and the onion with the cut sides facing down and fry them until the cut surfaces are well browned and the ginger is aromatic.

3 Then add the fish sauce, the seasoning powder and the crushed red pepper. Bring the contents of the pan to a boil, reduce the heat to low and let it simmer for about 20 minutes.

4 Strain the solids from the soup and stir in the lime juice.

5 Cook the ramen al dente, then drain and drain well. Then mix them with the sesame oil.

6 Spread the ramen in bowls and place the meat slices on top. Pour the hot broth over the dish and garnish with the ingredients for the garnish of your choice.

Ramen to go

for 2 servings

less than 30 minutes

easily

ingredients

40 grams of peas, frozen

60 grams of Chinese cabbage

60 grams of tofu

80 grams of ramen

½ teaspoon of salt

1 ½ teaspoon sesame oil, toasted

2 teaspoons of miso paste, dark

1 spring onion

1 carrot

4 shiitake mushrooms, dried

preparation

1 Pour boiling water over the shiitake mushrooms and let them steep for 10 minutes, then pour them off, squeeze them out and cut them into cubes.

2 Meanwhile, wash the Chinese cabbage and cut it into thin strips, peel the carrot and cut it into fine pencils, then dice the tofu about 1 centimeter in size.

3 Put the miso paste along with the salt and sesame oil in two preserving jars and stir everything together well. Then put the ramen, the carrots, the shitake cubes, the peas and the Chinese cabbage in the jars one after the other and seal them.

4 Wash and finely chop the spring onions and place them in separate containers.

5 To serve, pour 250 milliliters of boiling water into the jars, close the lids again and let the soup steep for 5 minutes. Then stir them well and garnish with the spring onions.

King prawn pot

for 4 servings

for 60 minutes

easily

ingredients

100 grams of sugar snap peas

125 grams of ramen

225 grams of king prawns

1.6 liters of vegetable stock

2 teaspoons of curry paste, red

1 tablespoon of lime juice

2 tablespoons of rapeseed oil

3 tablespoons of soy sauce

4 stalks of coriander

2 inches of ginger

1 pointed pepper, red

2 eggs

2 spring onions

2 carrots

preparation

1. Put the king prawns in a colander, wash them well, and let them thaw. Meanwhile, cook the eggs in a small saucepan for 10 minutes until they are hard. Peel the ginger and finely chop it. Wash and clean the vegetables thoroughly, then peel them. Cut the spring onion greens into fine rings, the carrots and pointed peppers into strips and halve the snow peas.

2. Heat some oil in a saucepan. Finely chop the white part of the spring onions and add it to the saucepan with the curry paste and chopped ginger. Then add the carrots and bell peppers and steam them a little. Then delete the contents of the pot with the vegetable stock and let the soup simmer for about 3 minutes.

3. Break the ramen into large pieces and add them to the soup along with the defrosted king prawns and the halved snow peas. Cook the ingredients for another 5 minutes.

4. Peel the eggs and cut them in half. Wash the cilantro thoroughly and shake it dry. Add the spring onion greens to the soup and taste with the soy sauce and lime juice.

5. Divide the soup into bowls and serve the dish with the halved eggs and the fresh coriander.

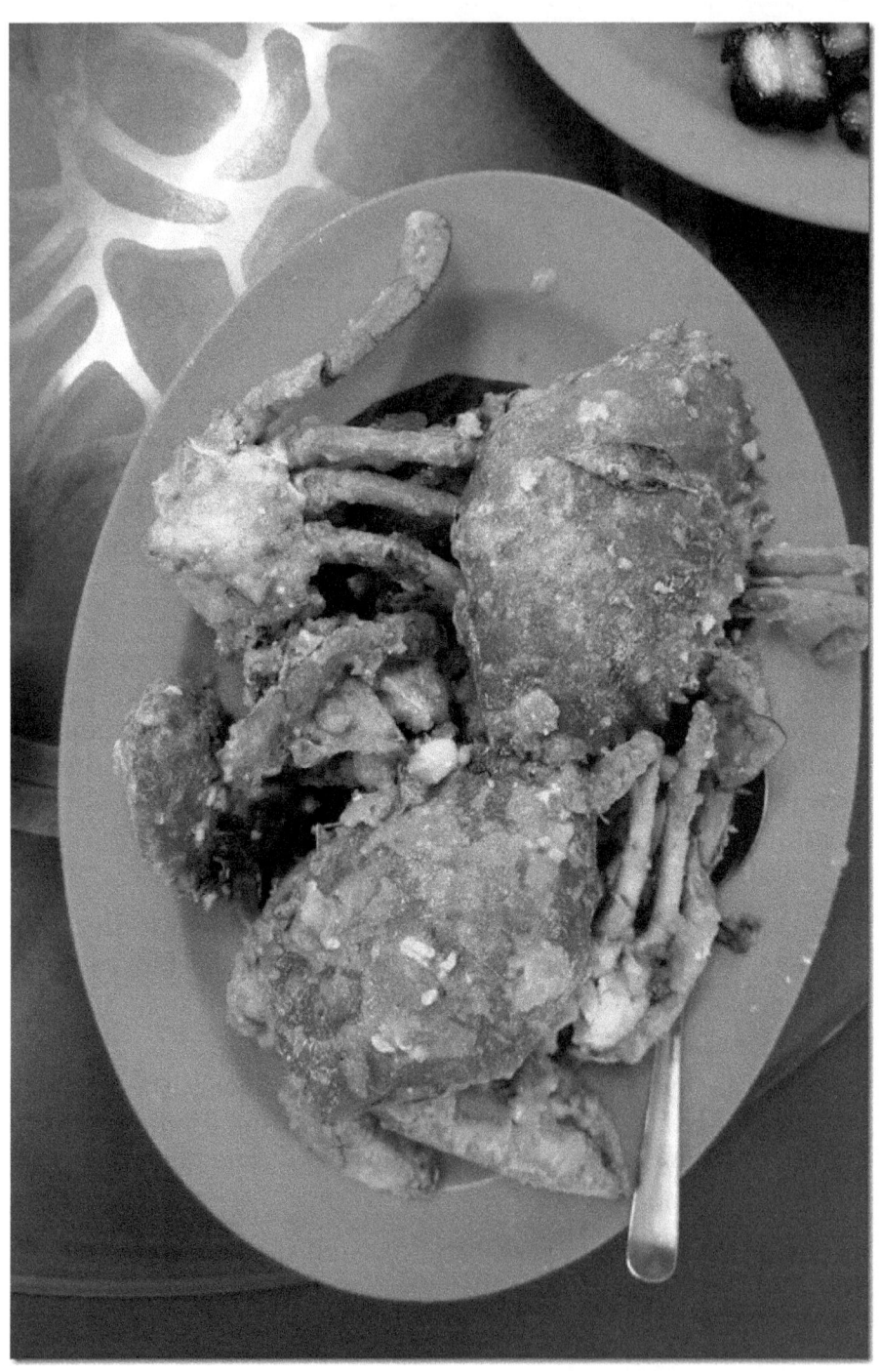

Beef ramen

for 4 servings

for 60 minutes

easily

ingredients

200 grams of ramen

500 grams of beef

600 milliliters of beef broth

1 teaspoon ginger, ground

1 tablespoon of vegetable oil

2 tablespoons of soy sauce

1 clove of garlic

1 onion Pak choi

preparation

1   Peel the clove of garlic and onion, then press the clove of garlic and finely chop the onion. Wash and clean the pak choi thoroughly and chop it up.

2 Heat some oil in a saucepan. Meanwhile, cut the beef into strips and fry them in the hot oil until they turn brown.

3 Add the stock, the ginger, the garlic and the onions to the saucepan and briefly bring to the boil. Then stir in the chopped pak choi, reduce the temperature, and let the soup simmer for a few minutes.

4 Add the ramen and simmer the soup for another 3 minutes. Stir in the oil and soy sauce and serve the soup with the meat.

Pork tenderloin and spinach ramen

for 4 servings

for 60 minutes

easily

ingredients

75 grams of baby spinach leaves

80 grams of mung bean sprouts

100 grams of mushrooms

250 grams of ramen

400 grams of pork tenderloin

2 teaspoons of vegetable broth

2 tablespoons of miso paste

2 tablespoons of rice wine

4 tablespoons of oil

4 tablespoons of soy sauce

3 centimeters of ginger

1 clove of garlic

1-2 chili peppers, red; 2 carrots

2 spring onions

4 eggs, size M

pepper

salt

preparation

1 Peel the ginger and garlic and chop both finely. Wash and clean the chili and spring onions and then cut both into fine rings. Pick the spinach and sprouts, place them in a colander, wash them thoroughly, and let them drain well. Clean and peel the carrots, then cut them into fine pencils. Clean the mushrooms and cut them into fine slices.

2 Heat 2 tablespoons of oil in a large saucepan. Add the chili, ginger and garlic and sauté everything for about 1 minute. Extinguish the contents of the pot with 1.2 liters of water and then stir in the broth. Boil everything and then add the miso paste, rice wine and soy sauce to taste.

3 Pat the meat dry with a paper towel. Then put it in the piece in the broth and let the meat sit on low heat for 20 minutes.

4 Meanwhile, cook the ramen al dente, pour them off and let them drain well. Put the eggs in a small saucepan and cook them until waxy for about 6 minutes, then pour them off, frighten them off, peel them and cut them in half.

5 Cut the meat into thin slices and arrange it in bowls together with the halved eggs, the vegetables and the ramen. Then spread the hot miso soup over it.

Pork ramen

for 4 servings

for 60 minutes

easily

ingredients

60 grams of ramen

120 grams of pork tenderloin

150 grams of radish, white

800 milliliters of vegetable broth

4 tablespoons soy sauce, light

5 tablespoons of mirin

½ organic lemon

1 carrot

1 clove of garlic

2 spring onions

6 shiitake mushrooms, dried

preparation

1 Cook the ramen, drain them in a colander, and let them drain well. Pour 200 milliliters of boiling water over the shiitake mushrooms and let them swell for 15 minutes. Then drain them off and catch the water in the process. Cut the mushrooms into strips.

2 Cut the meat into thin slices. Peel the carrot and radish and cut both into thin sticks. Wash the spring onions, clean them and cut their white part into pencils and the green part into thin rings. Rinse the lemon with hot water, dry it with a paper towel, and rub its peel thinly. Then squeeze out the lemon.

3 Boil the broth, peel the garlic and press it into the broth. Then stir in the mirin, mushroom water, soy sauce, lemon juice and lemon zest. Then add the meat and mushrooms and let the contents of the pan cook on medium heat for about 3 minutes.

4 Scatter the carrot, radish and onion sticks and let everything cook for another 3 minutes. Then stir in the ramen and let it get hot.

5 Spread the soup in bowls and garnish with the green of the spring onions.

Pork ramen soup

for 10 servings

for 30 minutes

easily

ingredients

50 grams of cabbage

50 grams of celery

65 grams of onions

150 grams of ramen

320 grams of pork, cooked

380 grams of asparagus

1 liter of water

½ teaspoon of garlic

¾ teaspoon of tarragon, dried

2 teaspoons parsley, fresh

1 tablespoon of olive oil

Cayenne pepper

preparation

1 Peel and chop the garlic and onion. Wash and clean the cabbage and celery and chop both. Wash the parsley, shake it dry, and chop it. Cut the cooked meat into cubes. Wash and peel the asparagus, and cut into pieces about two and a half centimeters long.

2 Fry the celery and onion in a large pan in oil until they both take on a soft consistency. Then add the garlic and cook for 1 more minute. Stir in the cayenne pepper, tarragon, cabbage, parsley, asparagus and water and bring to a boil.

3 Break the ramen and add them to the pan. Reduce the heat and simmer for to 5 minutes until the ramen is soft. Then add the diced meat and warm it up. Divide the soup into bowls for serving.

Summer soup

for 4 servings

for 60 minutes

easily

ingredients

100 grams of kimchi, cut into 3x3cm pieces

100 grams of radish, thinly sliced

250 grams of ramen

1 liter of chicken broth, unsalted

1 tablespoon of salt

1 tablespoon mustard powder

1 tablespoon of sugar

2 tablespoons rice vinegar

8 centimeters cucumber, thinly sliced

1 pear, quartered, cut into wedges

1 egg

8 large ice cubes

preparation

1 Put the chicken broth in a saucepan and heat it and season it with the vinegar, salt and sugar. Then let them cool and refrigerate for 1 hour.

2 Meanwhile, boil 4 liters of water in a large saucepan and cook the ramen in it for 5 minutes while stirring, pour them off, frighten them off and let them cool in ice water.

3 Boil the egg in a small saucepan for 9 minutes until it hardens, frighten it, then peel it and quarter it.

4   In a bowl, marinate the radish in 1 teaspoon of salt and 1 teaspoon of sugar.

5   Put all the ingredients in bowls and put them in the fridge.

6   Mix the mustard powder with 2 tablespoons of water to a paste 15 minutes before serving, let it stand for a moment.

7   Pour the paste on the dish, spread the ice cubes around the edges of the bowl and pour the cold broth over the top.

Bacon ramen

for 4 servings

90 minutes

ingredients

150 grams of ramen

500 grams of smoked bacon, mixed

250 milliliters rice wine or sherry, mild

1 teaspoon of five-spice powder

1 teaspoon of sugar

1 bunch of spring onions

2 inches of ginger

2 cloves of garlic

3 chili peppers

preparation

1. Wash and clean the spring onions thoroughly. Then cut the green into fine rings and let the white stand. Wash, clean, and halve the chili peppers lengthways. Peel the ginger and garlic and cut both into thin slices.

2   Put the white pieces of the spring onion together with the chili, ginger and garlic in a saucepan with 1 liter of water and cook everything for about 15

minutes. Then turn the heat to low and wait for the water to gentl billow. Then add the bacon with the spices, the rice wine and the sugar and let it cook for 30 minutes.

3   Cook the ramen al dente, then drain and rinse with cold water. Remove the bacon from the stock and cut it into fine slices. Add the noodles and the green onion rings to the stock, heat them up briefly and then divide everything into bowls. Garnish with the bacon slices to serve.

Tomato Ramen Soup

for 6 servings

less than 30 minutes

easily

ingredients

100 grams of ramen

450 grams of vegetables, frozen

500 grams of ground turkey

1 ½ liter of tomato juice

¼ teaspoon salt

¾ teaspoon of pepper

1 ½ teaspoon of sugar

1 bag of onion soup

preparation

1   In a large saucepan, cook the turkey on medium heat for 6 to 8 minutes until it is no longer pink and is slowly crumbling. Then add the onion soup mixture to the saucepan and stir it in. Season the whole thing with the pepper, 1 ½ teaspoon

ramen, the salt and the sugar. Deglaze the contents of the pot with the tomato juice and add the vegetables. Boil the whole thing briefly, reduce the heat and let everything simmer for about 5 minutes.

2 Break the ramen into small pieces and add them to the soup. Then cook the soup for another 3 to 5 minutes, stirring occasionally, until the ramen becomes soft.

3 Divide the soup into bowls and serve immediately.

lemon grass soup

for 2 servings

less than 30 minutes

easily

ingredients

100 grams of ramen

200 grams of baby spinach

500 milliliters of organic vegetable stock

1 tablespoon curry powder, mild

4 tablespoons of cashew nuts, salted, toasted

4 tablespoons of peanut oil

1 can of coconut milk (400 milliliters)

2 sticks of lemongrass

1 small chili pepper, red

1 small onion, red

salt

preparation

1. Cover and cook the pasta in boiling salted water. Pour the noodles off through a sieve after the cooking time, rinse them with cold water and let them drain well.

2. In the meantime, wash the chili pepper. Cut the lemongrass several times and put it in a saucepan with the broth, chili pepper, curry powder and coconut milk. Boil everything once and let it boil uncovered for about 2 minutes.

3. Coarsely chop the cashew nuts. Peel the onions and cut them into strips. Heat the oil in a large pan or wok and fry the cashew nuts, ramen and onion strips for about 4 minutes. Season the contents of the pan with salt.

4. Pick the spinach, wash it thoroughly and spin dry. Remove the chili pepper and lemongrass from the soup. Then add the spinach and let it cook for about 2 minutes. Add salt to the soup as you like.

5. Divide the soup into bowls, add the spinach and distribute the contents of the pan over it.

Banana split

for 2 servings

50 minutes

ingredients

25 grams of powdered sugar

65 grams of dark chocolate, finely chopped

100 grams of ramen

140 grams of flour

150 milliliters cream, 35%

150 milliliters of water

500 milliliters of coconut ice cream

1 teaspoon ginger, ground

1 teaspoon cinnamon, ground

1 egg; 2 bananas, halved lengthways;

Dulche de Leche

Desiccated coconut, toasted

salt

sugar

preparation

1   Preheat a Dutch oven with rapeseed oil to 175 degrees.

2   Mix the egg, flour, salt, water and sugar in a bowl. Dip the halved bananas in it so that they are completely coated with the batter. Put them in the Dutch oven to roast until they turn golden brown.

3 Put the ramen in the Dutch oven and deep-fry them until golden brown.

4 Mix the ginger with the powdered sugar then spread the mixture over the ramen.

5 Heat the cream over the stove and add the chocolate and cinnamon.

6 Now distribute the ingredients for the banana split on a plate and portion the coconut ice cream in balls. Finally, drizzle the dulce de leche and chocolate sauce over the dessert. Finally, garnish with the toasted coconut and serve immediately.

Butterscotch shards

for 2 servings

less than 30 minutes

easily

ingredients

125 grams of peanut butter

140 grams of ramen

170 grams of butterscotch chips

preparation

1 Line two baking sheets with parchment paper.

2 Cook the ramen al dente, then drain and drain well.

3 Place the butterscotch chips in a microwave-safe bowl and microwave them every 30 seconds.

4 Stir the peanut butter into the melted butterscotch chips. Add the ramen to the mixture and coat it completely.

5 Then use a tablespoon to spread small piles on the baking sheets and let them cool down so that they solidify. Then serve them straight away.

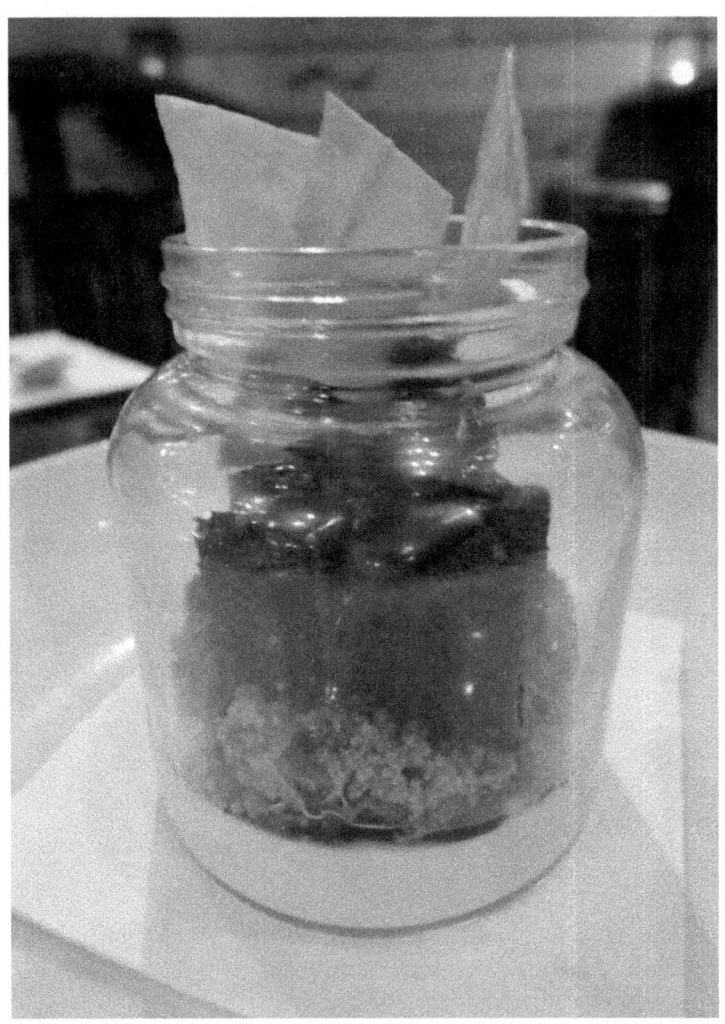

Ice cream ramen

for 4 servings

less than 30 minutes

easily

ingredients

35 grams of almonds, finely chopped

100 grams of ramen

150 grams of honey

2 tablespoons of butter

4 tablespoons of chocolate syrup

8 scoops of vanilla ice cream

Whipped cream

preparation

1   Melt the butter in a small pan and break the ramen into it. Fry them until they are crispy and they are brown.

2   Then reduce the heat of the pan and add the honey. Cook it while stirring until it starts to bubble and then add the almonds.

3   Put 2 scoops of vanilla ice cream in each bowl and distribute the contents of the pan over it.

4   Drizzle 1 tablespoon of chocolate syrup over each bowl and spread the whipped cream and serve dessert immediately.

Peanut Butter Bread

for 12 servings

90 minutes light

ingredients

100 grams of ramen

110 grams of peanuts, salted, chopped

110 grams of cottage cheese, low in fat

180 grams of sugar

240 grams of flour

75 milliliters of milk, low in fat

1 teaspoon of baking powder

1 teaspoon vanilla extract

1 ½ teaspoon nutmeg

1 tablespoon of margarine

2 tablespoons of butter

1 egg

preparation

1. Boil 300 milliliters of water, pull the saucepan off the stove and let the ramen soak in it for 2 minutes. Then drain them off and pat them dry with a paper towel. Then cut the pasta into pieces about two and a half centimeters long. Preheat the oven to 175 degrees.

2. Mix the baking powder, egg, cottage cheese, flour, milk, nutmeg, vanilla and sugar in a bowl using a hand mixer. Fold in the ramen and add half of the peanuts.

3. Grease a 2-liter casserole dish with margarine and pour the batter into it. Sprinkle it with the remaining peanuts and bake it in the preheated oven for about 50 to 60 minutes.

4. Cut the bread into 12 slices and serve with or without butter.

Peanut Butter Chocolate Ramen

for 24 servings

50 minutes light

ingredients

90 grams of rice grain

170 grams of peanut butter

170 grams of chocolate chips

6 tablespoons of butter, salted

200 grams of mini marshmallows

350 grams of ramen

1 teaspoon vanilla extract

preparation

1 Grease a 23 x 33 cm baking pan.

Melt butter in a large saucepan and stir in the marshmallows until they arealso melted and take on a smooth consistency. Stir in the vanilla extract and remove the pan from the stove.

3 Stir the peanut butter into the marshmallow mixture. Then fold in the ramen and rice cereal well until everything is thoroughly mixed.

4 Pour the mixture into the prepared baking pan and cool it for 15 minutes.

5 Melt the chocolate chips in the microwave until they have melted and spread them over the mixture in the baking pan. Finally cut these into 24 bars.

Honey and cinnamon ramen

for 2 servings

less than 30 minutes

easily

ingredients

200 grams of ramen

Strawberry sauce

honey

Whipped cream

cinnamon

sugar

preparation

1 Cook the ramen until tender, then drain and drain well - then let them cool in the refrigerator. Then place them on a plate and pour as much honey over it as you like.

2 Sprinkle the dessert with the cinnamon and sugar and spread the strawberry sauce on top.

3   Garnish the dessert with whipped cream and add a dash of strawberry sauce.

Crispy cherry ramen

for 2 servings

less than 30 minutes

easily

ingredients

100 grams of ramen

110 grams of pistachios, chopped

170 grams of cherries, dried, chopped

450 grams of almond slivers coated with vanilla

2 tablespoons of butter

preparation

1. Break the ramen into finer pieces. Melt butter in a large pan on medium to high heat and sauté the ramen with the cherries and pistachios. Then put the whole thing in a bowl to cool down.

2. Melt the coating on the almonds and pour the melted layer over the cooled ramen mixture. Gently stir everything and use a spoon to spread everything on a baking sheet lined with baking paper.

3 Let the dessert cool and set well, then store it in airtight containers at room temperature.

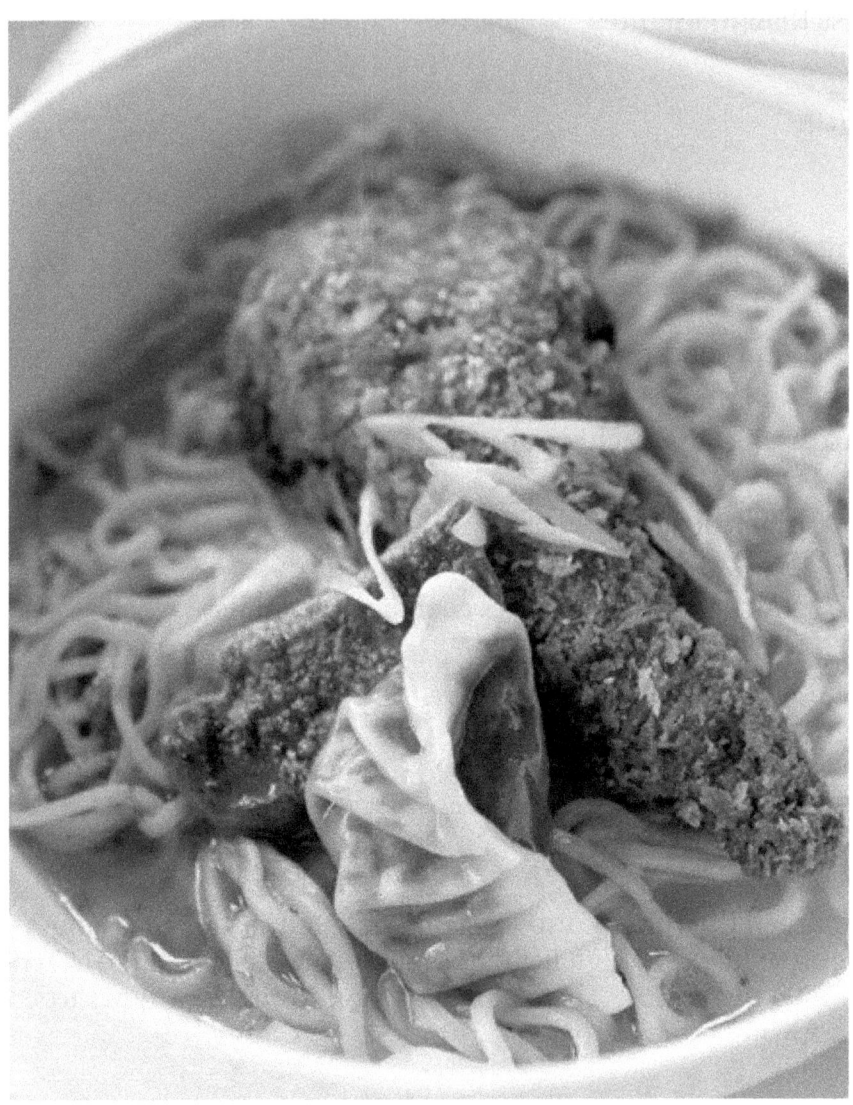

Cereal bites

for 10 servings

less than 30 minutes

easily

ingredients

60 grams of butter, melted

70 grams of almonds, sliced

80 grams of lingonberries, dried

100 grams of granola

150 grams of honey

170 grams of ramen

½ teaspoon cinnamon, ground

preparation

1   Preheat the oven to 175 degrees and line a baking sheet with parchment paper.

2   Break up the ramen and put them in a large bowl. Then add the almonds, granola, and dried cranberries.

3 Mix the butter, honey and cinnamon in a small bowl. Spread this mixture over the ramen mixture and stir everything well.

4 Spread the whole thing evenly on the baking sheet and bake it for 13 to 15 minutes in the preheated oven until it turns golden brown. Take the baking sheet out of the oven and let the muesli cool on a wire rack.

5 Cut it into large pieces and serve.

Peach ramen

for 2 servings

less than 30 minutes

easily

ingredients

45 grams of sugar, brown

50 grams of Kelloggs Frosties

100 grams of ramen

75 milliliters of peach juice, canned;

150 milliliters of cream; 1 can of peaches

preparation

1 Preheat the oven to 175 degrees.

2 Put all the ingredients - with the exception of the frosties - in a baking dish and mix them together. Make sure the ramen is covered with the rest of the ingredients.

3 Bake the whole thing in the preheated oven for about 5 minutes, spread the frosties over it and bake the dessert for another 5 minutes.

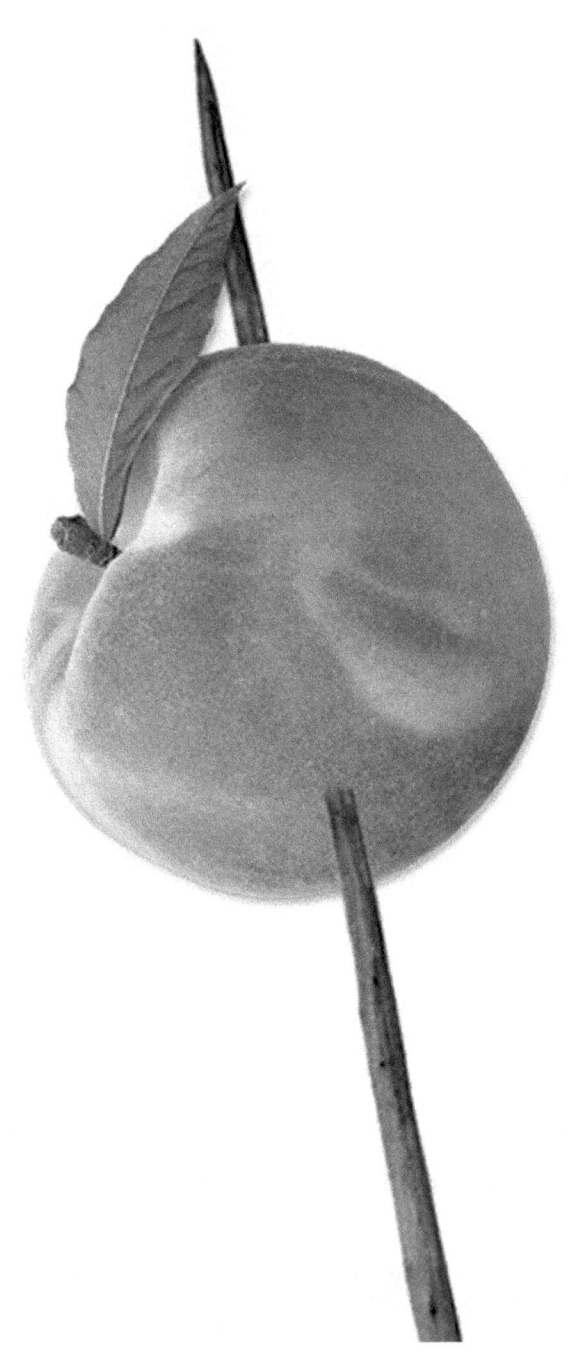

Ramen cookies

for 4 servings

less than 30 minutes

easily

ingredients

100 grams of white chocolate chips

200 grams of raisins

250 grams of ramen

2 tablespoons of butter

1 pack of M & Ms

preparation

1 Line your work surface with parchment paper.

2 Break the ramen into small pieces and transfer them to a bowl.

3   Melt the butter in a pan and heat it until it turns light brown. Then add the ramen until they too start to brown.

4 Melt the chocolate chips in the microwave and place them in a bowl with the M & Ms and raisins. Mix the whole thing with the ramen.

5 Use a tablespoon to place small heaps of the mixture on the baking paper and let it harden well.

Chocolate ramen

for 4 servings

for 60 minutes

easily

ingredients

100 grams of ramen

260 grams of dark chocolate

350 grams of condensed milk, sweetened

1 teaspoon butter

2 tablespoons of butter

powdered sugar

preparation

1   Break the ramen into small pieces and transfer them to a medium-sized bowl.

2   Melt the chocolate in a small saucepan and stir in the butter, condensed milk and vanilla.

3   Add the ramen to the pot and mix them with the chocolate mixture until they are completely coated.

4   Grease an 8 by 8 inch baking dish and pour in the chocolate mixture with the ramen. Let the whole thing harden for about 2 hours.

5   Cut the dessert into bite-sized pieces and serve.

Chocolate bar

for 4 servings

for 60 minutes

easily

ingredients

100 grams of ramen

170 grams of white chocolate chips

1 tablespoon butter, salted

1 ½ tablespoons of milk

preparation

1   Preheat the oven to 175 degrees.

2   Boil the ramen until al dente, drain them, rinse them with cold water, and then let them drain well.

3   Grease a baking sheet and spread the ramen evenly on it up to the edge. Then bake them in the preheated oven for around 30 to 40 minutes until they turn brown. Then take them out of the oven and let them cool down well.

4 Meanwhile, put the butter, milk and chocolate chips in a saucepan and melt everything over low heat, stirring constantly.

5 Pour the mixture from the pot over the cooled ramen and let it stand at room temperature for an hour.

6 Cut the whole thing into individual bars and serve them.

Chocolate vanilla ramen

for 4 servings

less than 30 minutes

easily

ingredients

100 grams of ramen

180 grams of sugar, brown

150 milliliters of chocolate syrup

300 milliliters of water

1 teaspoon vanilla

powdered sugar

Whipped cream

preparation

1   Boil the ramen until soft, add the brown sugar and let it steep for about 10 minutes, stirring occasionally. Then pour out the water.

2 Heat the contents of the pot over medium heat and add the chocolate syrup and vanilla, stirring occasionally. Let it sit for 5 minutes and then pull the pot off the stove again.

3 Before serving, place the dessert in the refrigerator for at least 1 hour and serve it with the powdered sugar and whipped cream.

Trail mix with honey

for 4 servings

for 30 minutes

easily

ingredients

45 grams of sugar, dark brown

100 grams of honey

115 grams of butter, melted

140 grams of almonds, finely chopped

160 grams of lingonberries, dried

170 grams of chocolate, white, cut into small pieces

300 grams of ramen

½ teaspoon of salt

1 teaspoon vanilla

1 teaspoon of cinnamon

preparation

1. Melt the butter in the microwave. Then put them in a bowl along with the honey, salt, cinnamon and brown sugar and stir everything together thoroughly.

2. Break the ramen into small pieces and add them to the bowl along with the almonds and cranberries. Mix everything together until everything is coated with the honey mixture. grease a baking sheet, spread the mixture on it and bake the whole thing for about 30 minutes in an oven at 160 ° degrees. Turn the mixture over once every 10 minutes.

3. Take the mixture out of the oven, let it sit for 5 minutes then stir again. Mix in the white chocolate pieces and transfer them into freezer-sealed bags. This will keep them at room temperature for about a week and in the freezer for several months.

Walnut pile

for 24 servings

70   minutes easily

Ingredients

40 grams of mini marshmallows

70 grams of walnuts, chopped

80 grams of lingonberries, dried

170 grams of ramen

255 grams of white chocolate chips

preparation

1   Line a baking sheet with parchment paper.

2   Break up the ramen and put them in a large bowl. Add the marshmallows, cranberries, and walnuts.

3   Melt the chocolate in the microwave every 30 seconds, stirring it over and over again. Then add the melted chocolate to the other ingredients in the bowl and mix everything together thoroughly.

4   Use a tablespoon to place 24 small piles on the parchment paper and let them set. Then serve them.

www.ingramcontent.com/pod-product-compliance
Lightning Source LLC
Chambersburg PA
CBHW071111030426
42336CB00013BA/2041